break through pain

SHINZEN YOUNG

break through pain

A Step-by-Step Mindfulness Meditation Program
for Transforming Chronic and Acute Pain

SOUNDS TRUE

Sounds True, Inc. Boulder, CO 80306
© 2004 Shinzen Young

SOUNDS TRUE is a trademark of Sounds True, Inc.

Published 2004
Printed in Korea

ISBN I-59179-199-5

Audio Learning Programs by Shinzen Young from Sounds True:
The Science of Enlightenment
Break through Pain
Break through Difficult Emotions
Meditation in the Zone
The Beginner's Guide to Meditation
Pain Relief

TABLE OF CONTENTS

Foreword

WHEN I FIRST MET Shinzen Young at a scientific conference in the winter of 1986, my psychological studies of altered states of consciousness had already gained me an international reputation as a scientific authority. In terms of intellectual knowledge, I was already an "expert" in meditation, but I had little personal experiential knowledge of meditation. I had received meditation instruction from a number of well-known teachers, but I had accepted that, when it came to meditation practice, I just did not have the necessary skills.

Then I heard Shinzen give his lecture on meditation, and the hairs stood up on the back of my neck. At some level deeper than intellect, a part of me was saying, "This man is speaking from direct experience, not book learning, and he knows what he's talking about!" I had listened to famous spiritual teachers over the years, but they had never touched me in this way.

Shinzen volunteered to teach meditation in early morning sessions for the rest of the conference. These sessions changed me from a person who believed he did not have the necessary talents for meditation to one who was not only learning the process, but enjoying it! Since that time, meditation has been a rewarding part of my daily life.

I have long been intrigued with Shinzen's work using mindfulness meditation to work with pain and suffering. Luckily, my interest has been primarily intellectual, for I hate pain and suffering, and do not want to personally test whether his methods work at high levels of pain! I have tested Shinzen's methods at relatively lower levels of pain and suffering, though, and they do work.

Suffering equals pain multiplied by resistance, Shinzen says. I recently experienced the effects of mindfulness and equanimity in reducing suffering. This story took place, interestingly enough, early in a ten-day retreat led by Shinzen that my wife and I were attending, just after Christmas of 2003. I had been experiencing, off and on, some "funny feelings" in my chest and body, including feeling faint when I got up in the middle of the night. My wife, Judy, is a nurse, and during the retreat when I told her about what I was feeling, she took my pulse and found it weak and irregular. A physician attending the retreat suggested that I go to a local hospital.

Half an hour later, I was in the emergency room, hooked up to all sorts of monitors, watching my irregular heartbeat on a monitor—sometimes very fast, sometimes skipping—and receiving injections to bring the fibrillations under control.

I managed to remain serene and calm throughout this experience. After all, I was at Shinzen's meditation retreat, practicing mindfulness and equanimity, and I saw no reason to stop the practice just because I was in a hospital. As Shinzen later remarked to me, the cosmos had transferred me from the basic meditation retreat to the advanced medication retreat.

Every once in a while that night, and the next couple of days in intensive care, as I observed my body sensations, thoughts, and internal imagery—the basic retreat practice—my thoughts and the corresponding images and body feelings would start to take off. "Oh my God, I'm in a hospital, my heart is skipping beats and acting crazy, my pulse is weak, I could die!" I kept observing the thoughts, images, and body feelings with as much attentiveness and equanimity as I could muster. In less than a minute, they would finish, and I would be calm and serene again, able to intelligently respond to what was needed.

Needless to say, I was impressed with myself, and with what I had learned from Shinzen. If there was ever a time to panic, being in a hospital with your heart acting up was a suitable occasion—and yet I was taking it all in stride. Suffering equals pain multiplied by resistance. I had enough meditative skill to have almost no resistance, so the psychological pain and resistance could not build up to any significant degree of suffering.

Current scientific research is finding that the age-old practice of mindfulness meditation can be very helpful for a variety of health challenges. As I know from experience, the technique can be difficult for many people to learn, so we are fortunate to have this book and CD of guided exercises by Shinzen, who I consider to be one of the world's foremost meditation teachers. After receiving his training and mastery under Eastern teachers, Shinzen systematically studied and experimented with ways of making meditation skills more relevant and easier to learn for modern Westerners.

The exercises presented here are one of his most successful applications: learning to greatly reduce and even eliminate the suffering that normally results from physical and psychological pain. Just about all of us will have to deal with such pain at least occasionally, if not frequently or chronically, so this book you hold in your hands is a great gift!

Charles Tart
Professor Emeritus of Psychology at UC Davis
Whose books include: the classic *Altered States of Consciousness; Mind Science: Meditation Training for Practical People;* and many others.

Introduction

IF YOU ARE reading these words, chances are you have a pain issue that remains unresolved. Perhaps you have tried other methods of relieving your pain, such as prescription medications or physical therapy, but have yet to find the relief that would allow you to live your life in a fully focused and present way, without being at the mercy of your discomfort.

As soon as pain arises in the body, the mind becomes preoccupied with how to get relief. If we can remove the cause of the pain or numb it with analgesics, well and good. But most people, at some time in their lives, face significant pain that they cannot escape. And hundreds of thousands of people, victims of disease or injury, must live each day in unavoidable and often excruciating pain.

If we cannot escape from the pain, must we then experience abject and meaningless suffering? Definitely not! There is an alternative, a way to escape not from but into the pain. We can apply Mindfulness Meditation to the pain. This is a way of focusing awareness on the pain and observing it with precision, while at the same time opening to it and dropping resistance. As you develop this skill, the pain causes less suffering and in many cases "breaks up" into a flow of pure energy. This may sound too good to be true, but it is a fact that has been independently discovered by thousands of individuals.

To be honest, it takes time, effort, and determination. On the other hand, growth of this skill "snowballs." That is to say, the more you practice, the faster you grow. Anyone can learn to develop this skill with regular practice, just as with sports or musical skills.

This approach to working with pain presents us with two challenges. The first challenge is conceptual: to understand the pain process in a new way, radically different from the usual. In the development of science, such fundamental changes in viewpoint are called paradigm shifts. Often it takes time and struggle before the new paradigm is accepted, but it is well worth it, because the new way of looking at things gives us so much power and clarity.

The second challenge is practical: to acquire the focusing skills and concentration needed to actually experience pain in a new, empowering way. This can be achieved through the systematic, sustained practice of mindfulness exercises.

Break Through Pain addresses both challenges. The book provides you with the necessary concepts, and the CD guides you in techniques for working with your pain. You can use these guided meditations frequently, even many times a day, if pain is a major issue in your life. Continue to use them day after day, until you develop the ability to meditate on your own.

This book is the culmination of many years of research and practice, and I am pleased to be able to share it with you to aid you in overcoming your own pain issues.

Many of the stories and examples in this book describe transcendence of intense or prolonged pain, but it is important to remember that the principles you will be learning here are very broad. You can use them to reduce or eliminate suffering due to any discomfort in your body, including minor aches and pains, or temporary discomfort due to tiredness, hunger, heat, cold, long hours standing or sitting, and so forth.

You can even apply what you learn here to sports activities and working out, by meditating on the body sensations that occur during such activities. With time, this can greatly increase your physical endurance and vastly deepen the euphoria sometimes known as "runner's high."

So, although I will frequently speak about working with "pain," in point of fact what I am really describing are strategies for working with any uncomfortable body sensation. This includes the body sensations of uncomfortable emotions, such as anger, fear, sadness, embarrassment, impatience, guilt, confusion, jealousy, and so on.

Learning the methods presented here will increase your freedom of choice regarding what you do to manage pain. These methods will work in conjunction with an aggressive drug-based pain management plan, to help with pain that gets past the medication. They can also be used as an alternative, to either reduce or eliminate the use of pain drugs.

After thirty years of using meditation practice to help people alleviate pain, I am still amazed at just how well these techniques work. People who could barely function before are often able to resume their lives as a result of regularly practicing meditation. The process is not always easy, but with intention and determination, you can make these techniques work for you.

CHAPTER
ONE

My Own Story

I CAME TO THE PRINCIPLES contained in this book through the practice of Buddhist meditation, and my own struggles in dealing with pain. I would like to share my story with you, so you will understand how my understanding of these techniques developed.

My earliest memories are of being physically "wimpy." I can remember that, if I stubbed my toe or was injured in any way, I would scream and cry. My mom tells me that I was what mothers call a difficult baby—very sensitive and hard to take care of in the first few years of life. I was easily upset, very finicky about foods, and so on. As a child, I did everything in my power to avoid physical discomfort. I would try any kind of trick or ruse I could think of to avoid going to the dentist or getting a shot. So I am not by nature a calm or patient person. In fact, I was probably drawn to meditation because I was the opposite type of person.

In junior high, I began to develop what was then an unusual interest: the study of Asian cultures. My best friend in junior high was a third-generation Japanese-American.

One Friday afternoon, my friend asked me if I would like to go with his family to see Japanese movies. I was not really interested, but I did not want to offend them, so I agreed. The first movie on the bill was a love story set in modern Japan, and I was completely bored. But the second one was a samurai movie, and I was mesmerized. It was set in eighteenth-century Japan, which seemed so incredibly exotic that it might as well have been another planet.

From that time on, every Friday I would go with them to see Japanese movies, and eventually they began to teach me the Japanese language. Then I discovered that there is an entire education system for Japanese-American children that runs parallel to the public schools, analogous to *hader*, or Hebrew school, for Jews. Classes met on weekdays when public school was over, and all day on Saturdays. I began to attend Japanese school, where I was the only non-Japanese student. My knowledge of Japanese was very limited when I enrolled, of course, but eventually I caught up. I graduated from Venice High School and Japanese language school in the same week. At Japanese school, I was chosen to be one of the valedictorians. I will never forget that scene: my parents sitting in the audience, listening proudly, but not understanding a single word.

I majored in Asian languages at UCLA, and enrolled in a study abroad program to go to Japan during my senior year. By that time, I could already speak, read, and write Japanese virtually like a native. During that year abroad, I had my first encounter with Buddhism. My initial interest was sparked by the fact that Buddhist temples resembled the sets of the samurai movies I had fallen in love with as a kid.

Then, during a visit to a temple, something happened that had a deep impact on me: A monk reached out and took my hand, and that simple gesture was a seminal moment for me. I thought, "These people have a secret, and they would be happy to share it, but they are not going to push it on me. Rather, there is an outstretched hand here."

When I returned to UCLA for graduation, I spoke to my favorite professor about Buddhism and Buddhist culture, and he suggested that I enter the University of Wisconsin's Ph.D. program in Buddhist studies. At this point, during the culture shift brought about by the Vietnam War, government money was being poured into Buddhist studies because we needed to have the Buddhists on our side in Southeast

Asia. I ended up with a large government grant that allowed me to attend graduate school with an emphasis in Buddhist studies.

When I completed my coursework, the university sent me back to Japan. I was supposed to do research on the Shingon School of Mount Koya. Shingon is a distinct school of Japanese Buddhism, and involves practices somewhat similar to those of Tibet. At that time, it had never been studied by a Westerner. My plan was to become the sole expert in the Western world on this school of Buddhism, but the monks in residence at Mount Koya would not teach me anything because I was merely intellectually curious. They said, "If you want to learn about Buddhism, you have to practice."

That was the beginning of my meditation career. It was very difficult at first, because I was asked to sit bolt upright and with crossed legs for an hour without moving. Very quickly, my only focus was on the physical pain caused by sitting. By the end of the hour, I would be devastated, holding on for dear life. I would clench my fists as my whole body shook. Often I was on the verge of tears, in agony from the physical discomfort of keeping the body motionless for that long.

But I respected the people who were teaching me, and they said, "This is the time-honored way," so I continued to try. Every sit ended up feeling like a torture session. The monks gave me a breath meditation, similar to the one I present on Track Five of this integrated book/CD. The breath focus did help somewhat, but very quickly, I was back in pain and all my reactions to the pain.

After a number of months of daily practice, I started to get a little bit of concentration, and was able to hold my attention without distraction, which felt really good. My breath slowed down naturally, and I noticed that my internal talk was not as loud. Although I did not notice it at the time, in retrospect, I realize that not only did my internal talk quiet down, but my mental images and emotional reactions to the pain were also reduced. Because, like most people, I was centered on self-talk, what I initially noticed most prominently was a quieting of the "internal dialogue." That was my initial breakthrough.

After a few months, it was suggested that I attend a *sesshin* at a Zen Temple. In Japanese, sesshin refers to a week-long intensive meditation retreat in the Zen tradition. Well, the first sit felt great; the second sit felt great; the third sit started to hurt a little. By the fourth sit, I realized I was in trouble. There were going to be about twenty such half-hour sits each day, and this was only the first day of the week!

Things got worse and worse. By the last sit of the last day, my mind was becoming grossly distorted by the pain; I was losing contact with reality and having paranoid ideas that the monks were making the sits longer just to torture me, a foreigner. The pain was literally driving me insane. During that last sit, my whole body shook violently, and I realized I was on the verge of tears. I started to scream to myself, inwardly, "You're not a baby, don't cry. You're not a baby, don't cry."

Then suddenly, out of nowhere, everything just dissolved. The pain turned into waves of energy. My internal conversation vanished into deep quiet, and my mental screen dissolved into vibrant white light. My body completely relaxed; the pain was simply energy. At that moment, I experienced a kind of restfulness of soul unlike anything I had known in this life. This experience continued for ten or fifteen minutes, then the bell rang, and the sesshin was over. But those few minutes changed me forever.

That next winter, I entered a hundred-day, isolated training on Mount Koya. One of the masters there finally offered to teach me, and gave me the Buddhist name Shinzen. "We'll start at the winter solstice," he said. "The training will last one hundred days, it will be in isolation, and you'll have no source of heat, but if you want to do the traditional training, this is the way it's done."

There was an added surprise when I actually started this training: It turned out that, three times a day, I was expected to go to a wooden cistern, break through the ice on top, fill a wooden bucket, and pour the freezing water over myself. This was required before each of the meditation periods.

On day three, I was pouring the water over my head and attempting to dry myself, and the towel was freezing in my hands. At that moment, I had an epiphany. I had noticed during the first three days that every time my mind wandered, my sense of suffering increased, and every time I regained my concentration, my sense of suffering was diminished. It became crystal clear to me that I had only three choices: Either I would spend the next ninety-seven days in abject misery, or I would give up and return to America, or I would spend those ninety-seven days in a concentrated state, twenty-four hours a day. There was no fourth option. I did not want to give up, and I certainly did not want to spend ninety-seven days in misery, so I vowed to do my best to stay in a continuous concentrated state.

My only source of solace was this state of concentration. As I see it now, this retreat in isolation was a hundred-day biofeedback device to assure unbroken concentrative work. I went in one person and I came out a different person. It was intense, but it was a small price to pay for a new life, or more accurately, a new kind of life. From the time I finished the training until this very moment, the concentrated state has never entirely left.

After I completed my hundred-day training, I stayed on in Japan for two more years. During that time, I continued to train at Mount Koya in the Shingon tradition, as well as attend Zen retreats in Kyoto, the old capital of Japan.

During one of those Zen retreats, I met someone who fundamentally changed the direction of my life. The retreat was about to begin, and I was already seated in the meditation hall, when I noticed that there was another foreigner present—and not just a foreigner, but a Roman Catholic priest. When he came into the meditation hall I thought, "How strange, a Catholic priest at a Zen retreat. He sure doesn't know what he's in for!" but then he sat down in perfect lotus posture, and immediately entered what was obviously a deep meditative state. He looked like a seasoned Zen monk.

During one of the break periods, I went up to him and introduced myself. This man who had piqued my curiosity turned out to be Father William Johnston, a Christian missionary from Ireland who indeed had practiced Zen meditation for several decades.

Growing up Jewish, I had little contact with the Christian world, and virtually no contact with Catholicism. Eventually Father Bill and I became good friends, and through him I came to a startling realization: Prior to meeting him, I had assumed that the special states of consciousness I was experiencing in Buddhist meditation were unique to Buddhism. Through my conversations with Father Johnston I came to realize that Buddhist meditation is just one representative of a broad universal experience found within all religions, as well as within secular contexts. This put my Buddhist experience within a much larger, more universal framework.

I began to avidly study the mystics and meditators of the Christian, Islamic, Taoist, Hindu, and Jewish traditions. I was captivated by the medieval Christian text known as *The Cloud of Unknowing* and the works of St. Teresa of Avila, Jalal-uddin Rumi, Isaac Luria, Thomas Merton, and many others. In particular, I was amazed and delighted to discover that, although meditation is not central to Judaism, as it is to Buddhism, there had been a Jewish meditative tradition, and that there was an entire technical vocabulary in Hebrew that described the very experiences I had encountered while doing Buddhist practice!

From that time on, I have viewed meditative states not as a "Buddhist thing" but as a universal human experience. Shortly before I was to leave Japan, I had a final meeting with Father Johnston. He was very excited about an article he had read regarding scientists who were studying meditative states. Father Johnston was a member of the Jesuits, an order which historically drew from the intellectual elite of Catholic Europe, a tradition that has continued to this day. The idea that Western science could perhaps validate Christian and Buddhist experience was intellectually riveting for him, and for me, too.

I thought to myself, "I'm going back to the Western world, where science originated. Maybe I should use this as an opportunity to learn something about science." Shortly after my return to the United States, I participated in a retreat at the International Buddhist Meditation Center in Los Angeles with Dr. Thich Thien-an, a Vietnamese monk I had known before I went to Japan. I asked him if he had heard that scientists were studying meditation. As Dr. Thien-an was himself an educator and an intellectual, I thought he would be interested in such topics. In fact, he told me that not only did he know about this research, but that three of the primary researchers were at that very retreat. Talk about serendipity!

After the retreat, I introduced myself to the researchers. This was the beginning of a significant new direction in my life. It occurred to me that often in history, two areas of knowledge which developed independently at some point have found a common ground, cross-fertilized one another, and produced a radically new direction in human knowledge. Looking at the big picture, it seemed to me that, in the broad sweep of human history, the two most impressive discoveries are the external science of the West and the internal science of the East. "What a weird and wonderful hybrid child might be born of their cross-fertilization," I thought. From this coming together of East and West, perhaps a whole new direction in human understanding and a whole new technology for human improvement could be evolved.

I have spent the last three decades exploring that possibility. But, initially, I had one enormous problem: I had failed all my math and science classes in high school and college. I suffered from math phobia, and had a dismal academic record in the sciences. Fortunately, though, I now had meditation skills: I had concentration abilities; I had some ability to listen to my negative tapes without believing them; I had some ability to observe my emotions without being distorted by them. When the belief that I would fail arose, I could often observe the internal talk, the mental images, and the emotional feelings of this belief without buying into them. The equanimity and concentration power I had gained through meditation training allowed me to overcome the limiting influence of the past and actually become quite accomplished in the areas of math and science. In fact, I eventually went on to teach such subjects at the college level.

In turn, my scientific studies have dramatically influenced the way I teach meditation. I attempt to bring the spirit of rigor, quantification, and experimentalism that characterizes Western science into my teaching of Buddhist meditation. The results have been deeply and powerfully satisfying.

I set myself a life goal: to apply what I learned in math and science to teaching meditation in the attempt to find better ways to teach mindfulness practice based on the spirit and methods of Western science. Of course, I am not so arrogant as to think that I can totally redesign the methods passed down to us for centuries and millennia, but I do think it is possible to make significant improvements, and furthermore to describe the entire process in the universal secular vocabulary of science, making it accessible to anyone in the contemporary world.

After I returned from Japan, I lived at the temple of Dr. Thich Thien-an for many years, dividing my time equally between the practice of my own meditation and the study of science. I never officially proclaimed myself a meditation teacher. Rather, because people found my approaches contemporary and clear, word spread, and more people began to study meditation with me.

Among those students were people with physical pain issues. I began to work with them, knowing from my own experience the steps one must go through to transcend and eventually transmute pain. I became known as someone who could explain mystical states, but also as someone who knew about the nuts and bolts of dealing with physical discomfort.

Eventually, in 1982, I opened my own center in the Korea Town area of Los Angeles, with a small community of residents who meditated together. Each morning, during our group meditation, I would give interviews with the residents, discussing their practice. Traditionally in such interviews, the student and the teacher discuss the practice, and then the student is sent back to the cushion to implement the results of that discussion, but I started to experiment with a somewhat different approach: I would sit in front of the students as they meditated for an hour or more. At the beginning of the session, I would give them a meditation procedure, have them practice it, and then three of four minutes later query them about what they had experienced. Based on what they reported, I would give them feedback in various forms. I might say, "The best thing to do is to continue what you're doing," or, "Let's make the following modification to what you're doing," and so forth, depending on what they had reported. A few minutes later, I'd query them again, modifying the procedure if needed, offer interpretation or encouragement, share my own experiences with them, or give them a range of choices as to what we might explore next.

The first thing I discovered about this "interactive" method is that it was much more effective than the standard "Here's the teaching, there's the cushion, now do it" approach. In the early stages of meditation practice, a lot of time is typically spent just spinning one's wheels; beginning students are often lost in daydreams, preoccupations, sleepiness, confusion, and so on. By way of contrast, if they have a meditation coach sitting in front of them, the internal distractions are greatly diminished. They are much more likely to be focused on their procedure for the entire sitting time. After experiencing what a "quality sit" is like under such guidance, they are better able to replicate it when sitting alone.

The other discovery I made was that the students' perception of time was dramatically altered though this interactive process. They were able to work for long periods without perceiving that much time had passed. Thus, this method of interactive guidance allows students to do extended practice without it seeming burdensome.

Finally, and most importantly, I found that this method was an optimizing procedure. Here is what I mean by that: I believe that, literally every minute, Nature is presenting us with windows of opportunity for transcendence. The problem is that most people don't recognize them, let alone make use of them. When I interactively guide a student, I share my expertise. I point out those windows of opportunity, and suggest ways to utilize them.

Even to this day, after years of exploring this process, I still do an analysis after each session to see what worked and what didn't work. I've thus been able to continuously hone the procedure into a detailed algorithm of transcendence. The techniques I give you on the CD represent the broad outline of that algorithm.

CHAPTER
TWO

The Practice of Meditation

DEALING WITH PAIN from illness or injury becomes a major issue for most people sometime in their lives. Indeed, for millions of chronic pain victims, it is *the* issue every moment of their lives. But there is a way to break through this pain through the practice of Mindfulness Meditation.

More importantly, when you break through pain in this way, you get a sense of being empowered and even nurtured by it—strange as that may sound. Thus, meditation is not merely a way to manage pain, but actually allows you to experience pain as deeply meaningful in the sense of contributing to psychological and spiritual growth.

We might say that there is good news and bad news regarding the fact that you have a pain issue: The bad news is that you have a pain issue. The good news is that techniques such as those I will describe are available to deal with it. The best news is that those techniques do not just affect your relationship to the pain; they affect your entire life. In learning them, you will be learning to develop the focusing power of your own mind. The focusing power of your own mind is the single most important tool that you have in this life.

It is good to understand these techniques in their broad historical context. The approach presented here is derived from the Mindfulness tradition, which goes back to the original discoveries of the Buddha some 2,500 years ago, but the techniques themselves are completely removed from the cultural background and doctrinal system of Buddhism. For decades, they have been used in Western clinical settings without any religious connotation. When you use these techniques, you will never be asked to do anything other than the following three things: observe precisely, have equanimity, and be sensitive to how things change. Certainly, no one could have any objection to being alert and self-accepting.

So, although these techniques are derived from the discoveries of the Buddha, they are being presented here in a broader context. If you have your own religious or philosophical system, you can be confident that these teachings will not be in conflict with your beliefs.

WHAT IS MEDITATION?

Everybody has had meditative experiences, although you may not have thought of them that way at the time. Many people hold stereotypes about what it means to meditate, but I prefer to define meditative states in terms of the experiences of daily life. If you think about an activity in your life that has been meaningful to you, you will probably remember times when you were very focused and "present" during that activity, and other times when you were scattered and unfocused. Whatever activity you were engaged in—running, playing the guitar, making love—recall how, at the times when you were completely present and focused, the activity was incomparably more fulfilling. Everyone is aware of these fluctuations in our degree of presentness or focus in daily life. In fact, if you reflect back on your life, you may remember a few very significant times when you became extraordinarily focused. This state of extraordinary focus generally takes place under one of two circumstances: Sometimes it occurs when you are particularly relaxed—perhaps walking in the forest alone, or after a particularly meaningful experience of making love, for example—and you are able to enter a state of extreme presence and deep quiet.

The other circumstance under which this state of extraordinary focus can occur is at the opposite end of the spectrum, in dangerous, even life-threatening situations: you are about to be involved in a car accident; you think you are going to drown; you are physically accosted. At those moments, you find that time slows down, you are peaceful, and you are extremely present and focused on what is happening, and thus able to deal with the situation more effectively, both subjectively and objectively.

Everyone acknowledges fluctuations in their day-to-day level of focus, and many people have had occasional experiences of extraordinary focus. If asked, most people would agree that, in the focused state, life is deeper and more fulfilling.

However, what few people realize is that the focused state is something that can be cultivated through systematic practice. Thus, your concentration level does not have to be controlled by day-to-day, random fluctuations, and you do not need to wait for extreme or unusual conditions to "enter the zone"; your baseline of presence and focus can be elevated through systematic practice. Therefore, both in terms of your subjective world and your objective performance, the entire scale at which you live your life can be elevated, across the board.

That focus can be cultivated is one of the most significant discoveries that the human species has made. The metaphor that I like to use is that it is very much like exercising a muscle. If you think about the process of physical exercise, what is involved? You have to learn a certain procedure for doing the exercise so that it is effective, and you do not harm yourself; you have to exercise on a regular basis; you have to be willing to put some effort into it; and you have to make it part of your daily regimen. If you are willing to do these things, you can strengthen your muscles. This improved physical strength is then always available for your life activities.

What we might refer to as concentration strength can also be improved through exercise. The process is similar to that of strengthening your muscles. You need instruction in certain procedures, you need to do the procedures on a regular basis, you need to keep practicing for the long term, and you need to maintain a commitment to the practice. As a result, your concentration power can be permanently strengthened.

Once this has occurred, all of the activities you engage in are improved. Every aspect of your life is affected, because every aspect of your life depends on focus. One could say that focus is the most fundamental of human skills.

The notion of extending the human lifespan is an archetypal theme in many cultures. For example, in the West, we have the legend of the Fountain of Youth, while in the East there is the notion of internal alchemy. Suppose I were to tell you that I had a procedure such that, if you practiced it for half an hour each day, it would add one hundred years to your life, guaranteed. You would undoubtedly think that was a terrific idea. Of course, no such procedure exists. However, there is a process—namely, meditation—that will dramatically expand the *scale* of each moment of your life. It is certainly possible to double the baseline of your concentration in daily life. Living each moment with twice as much focus means living each moment twice as big, twice as deep. Then, even if you were to live only sixty years, the total richness of your life would be the equivalent of 120 years.

What all meditation systems around the world have in common is that they show you how to develop an extraordinary degree of focus, and therefore allow you to live your life on an expanded scale.

There is no aspect of human life to which meditation skills cannot be applied. Actually, that is why a lot of people have difficulty understanding meditation. They ask, "What is it good for?" not realizing that it is good for everything! It will allow you to be more present in your interactions with other people, to gain a greater understanding of yourself through introspection, and to pursue your spiritual path more effectively. It will increase creativity and intellectual capacity, allow you to experience physical and emotional discomfort with less suffering, to experience physical and emotional pleasure with heightened fulfillment, and to resist negative urges. Success in any human endeavor is predicated upon one's ability to focus. Therefore, it makes sense that focus as an independent skill should be systematically taught in school. But in point of fact, not only is it not taught, it is not even mentioned!

Concerning the systematic cultivation of focus, there are a number of stereotypes and misconceptions. One misconception is that there is a single "meditative state." In fact, the meditative states represent a continuum, from light states of concentration that most people have experienced, to special states of profound absorption. Over the months and years that you practice meditation, one of the dimensions in which you will grow is the dimension of depth. By that, I mean you will come to experience deeper and deeper states along this continuum.

In addition to the dimension of depth, there is a second dimension in which meditation grows, which you can think of as breadth. By breadth, I mean that the meditative state spreads to encompass more and more complex activities of ordinary life. A common misconception about meditation is that it is a state you enter only while you are sitting still. At first, it may be that meditation is simply one of your life activities; at some point, though, a figure-ground reversal takes place. Instead of meditation being one of the activities in which you engage in daily life, daily life is contained within your meditative state. You are simply there, all the time.

An appropriate metaphor here is the process of learning to drive a car. When you first learn how to drive, all you can do is keep track of what you need to drive the car; you cannot do anything else, because the new skills demand so much of your attention. But when those skills have been completely internalized, you can go onto a road, and eventually onto the chaos of the freeway.

In the same way, when you first begin to meditate, indeed, you may be barely able to achieve a little concentration while sitting still, but with practice, the skills become internalized. At first, you may be able to maintain that state when standing up, and then when walking around. After more practice, you can engage in simple activities, such as cleaning the house, and still maintain your meditative state. Eventually, you will be able to carry on conversations, drive your car, and even fill out your tax forms without ever leaving the meditative state.

Formal sitting is to meditation as playing scales is to music. Even great musicians still play scales, but scales are not the purpose of music. In the same way, even experienced meditators still do formal sitting practice, but formal sitting practice is not the goal of meditation. The concert is the goal of music practice; living one's life fully is the goal of the meditation practice.

Let me make more tangible what I mean by the meditative state. Take some simple activity, like washing the dishes. In the usual, non-meditative state, your mind will go to the past, go to the future, go to fantasy; in other words, your attention is scattered. There is nothing intrinsically wrong with being scattered, but it would be nice to at least have the *option* of doing things differently.

Let's say you would like to "just wash the dishes." What does that mean in terms of tangible sensory experience? It means that your attention goes only to what is relevant to washing the dishes. That involves three sensory experiences: the body sensations of touching the dishes and water, the visual impressions of the washing process, and the sounds made by the water and the dishes. If you fully focus on these, there is no room left in consciousness for memory, planning, and fantasy. You have united or merged with the activity of dishwashing. This ordinary experience has now become ecstatic and extraordinary.

A third stereotype about meditation is that it involves a limiting of your awareness, a narrowing of the focus. That is entirely incorrect. Meditation is a limiting only in the sense that it is a focusing on exactly what is relevant to a certain situation, but what is relevant to a certain situation may be quite broad. For example, when you interact with another human being, what is relevant to that situation? When they speak, what is relevant is that you experience their entire being—their physical appearance and the sound of their voice. When you speak, what is relevant is that you fully manifest your personality. The problem is, when we have human interactions, we are often quite scattered into what is irrelevant, and therefore unable to fully experience the other person, and also unable to fully manifest our own personalities.

I hope these examples help make a little more tangible the relevance of meditative states to ordinary life.

MEDITATION AND THE FIXATION WITH THINKING

As I have mentioned, the mind's preoccupation with things that are irrelevant to the task at hand is a major challenge to achieving a meditative state.

The great majority of human beings are literally addicted to thinking. Even the most wretched substance abuser can go a few hours between "fixes," but most human beings cannot abide even for a few seconds without some sort of "thought fix." If there is nothing significant to think about, we fill the void with fantasy, trivia, and internal music.

Simply stated, meditation breaks the addiction to thinking. One is then in a highly desirable situation: When you want to have a complete experience of hearing and feeling (for example, as you listen to music), you can do so without being compulsively pulled into thoughts which are not relevant to the music. When you want to have a complete experience of tasting and feeling, as when enjoying a bite of food, you can likewise do so. On the other hand, when it is appropriate to think, you find that your thinking abilities are vastly improved. This improvement in thinking stems from two causes. The first is easy to understand. The second is a little subtle.

Breaking the compulsion to think simply means that the thinking process is no longer scattered by distracting forces. So, when you turn your mind to some topic, you can penetrate that topic with great clarity and vigor. To draw a metaphor from the physical world, when thinking is no longer at the mercy of scattering forces, it becomes like a penetrating beam of coherent laser light. I am quite convinced that this aspect of meditation makes a person a better student and problem-solver, and actually elevates one's I.Q.

But there is a more subtle way in which meditation improves one's thinking abilities. Here, once again, a metaphor may be helpful: When a person works through a compulsive eating problem, they certainly do not stop eating. In point of fact, they are able to taste and appreciate their food in an entirely new way. Analogously, when a person works through the compulsive need to have answers, the answers begin to come in an entirely new way. The thinking process becomes spontaneous and intuitive. Personal and spiritual insights well up effortlessly of their own. At this point, there is no need to stop the thought process in order to be in a state of meditation, because the thought process itself has returned to being part of the effortless flow of Nature. Because this mode of thinking is so dramatically different from ordinary congealed thought, each of the major spiritual traditions has a technical term for it. In Christianity it is called sophia, in Judaism, chochma, and in Buddhism, prajña.

Meditation offers two basic strategies for breaking our addiction to thought: The first is to constantly let go of distractions and return to some focus; for example, the breath or a mantra. The second is to allow the thought to "do its thing," but to carefully observe it with detachment.

In order to better understand the thought process and how it relates to meditation, you can do an experiment: Sit down and take a minute to let your body settle. After you settle in, pay close attention to your thinking process. Your thoughts will tend to come either as internal talking, internal imaging, or both at the same time. The talking may be words, phrases, or whole sentences. You may hear your own voice, or the voices of other people. The images may be quite clear and vision-like, or just vague impressions of objects, faces, and situations. Take a hands-off attitude with regard to this sequence of internal dialogues and mind's-eye imagery. Give it permission to come and go, to start and stop, to speed up and slow down as it wishes. But be very alert! Every few seconds, there will be new words or sentences. Every few seconds, the pictures will change, perhaps slightly, perhaps totally.

In order to help you be precise and matter-of-fact about this process, do the following: Each time you begin to think in words or sentences, say out loud, "Talk." Each time you get new pictures, say out loud, "Image." If you get both at the same time, say, "Talk and image." The words and the images may continue as you note them, or they may immediately die away. Either case is okay. The only goal is to be very clear at any given moment whether you are thinking in words, images, or both.

After a while, if your concentration is good, you may feel like dropping the spoken labels. You can then either say the labels to yourself, or just be directly aware of the categories without attaching labels. But as soon as you get spaced out or caught up, immediately reinstate the spoken labels. Of course, mentally labeling your thoughts is itself a kind of thought. However, you will not be confused if you remember this simple rule: Do not label the labels! Consider them to be a special category of artificial thought that helps you keep track of natural thought.

You may experience periods of time during which there is no thought, and the mind is quiet and peaceful. Paradoxically, when we take a hands-off attitude toward thought, not trying to suppress it, but just observing it, the mind sometimes spontaneously stops on its own for a period of time.

Another possibility is that you may be thinking, but the thoughts are not in clear words or images. It is more like a background hum, the gears of the mind turning somewhere deep down, but you are not sure (or have only a vague sense) of the topic. We might call this kind of thinking subtle processing. It is the preconscious or subconscious activity out of which the conscious "talking" and "imaging" arises moment by moment. Because it is a spreading wave of many rapid and fleeting subconscious associations, it is usually neither possible nor necessary to know its precise content. To try to do so would be like trying to keep track of the individual droplets of water in a cloud. We can, however, observe the macroscopic waveform of the cloud as a whole, how it speeds up, slows down, spreads, and collapses. The concept of subtle processing may be a little difficult to grasp. Basically think of it this way: If your mind is not perfectly still, but neither can you identify the thoughts in terms of clear words or images, then you are experiencing subtle processing.

Usually, when a person first begins to meditate, they are acutely aware of the surface conscious thoughts such as the ones that occur in clear images and words, especially words. As the thinking process becomes less driven, one also becomes aware of intervals of quiet and subtle processing. The mind is a "fractal" structure in nature, like vegetation. After the big trees have been cut down, one becomes aware of both clear patches and the finer underbrush.

The subtle processing could also be described as embryonic thought or preconscious processing. Although it is too fleeting to observe its specific content, one can observe its activation level—how it speeds up, slows down, gets more intense, gets less intense—moment by moment. As one observes the wave qualities of this subtle processing, giving it permission to "do its thing," it becomes unblocked and fluid.

When this happens, the deep levels of processing become energized and undulatory. This produces two desirable effects: First, it frees up our intuitive faculty. New insights well up directly from the fluid matrix of subtle processing, without having to be first processed at the conscious level. Second, the subtle processing tends to be continuous. In that sense, it is easier to observe than the words and images, which tend to be sporadic and fleeting. One can rest awareness continuously on the flow of subtle processing. This allows you to experience the wave-like, vibratory nature of thought.

DIVIDE AND CONQUER

The underlying theme of Mindfulness Meditation is the concept of "divide and conquer." As you will see, this skill is particularly important in working with pain. Here is the basic idea: if an experience is overwhelming you, break it up into its parts, and keep track of them as they arise moment by moment. Often, the separate parts are quite manageable individually, hence the aggregate experience loses its power to overwhelm you.

A phenomenon cannot overwhelm you as long as you can divide it into manageable parts. By separating experience into parts, we divide its gripping power. A hundred-pound rock represents a crushing weight. Two fifty-pound rocks can be handled, albeit with effort.

This divide-and-conquer principle can be applied to any type of sensory experience. For example, the gripping power of your thoughts is greatly reduced by deconstructing thought into internal talk and mental image. The gripping power of body sensation is greatly reduced by dividing it into separate flavors—physical touch, emotional feel, and so forth—and then subdividing the flavors into locations.

The expression "divide and conquer" originated with the Romans, but here, I am using it in a somewhat different sense. We certainly are not trying to conquer thought or pain, or any other sensory phenomenon, for that matter. What gets conquered is the driven-ness, fixation, and unconsciousness that pervade our sensory experience.

When we conquer these, we conquer internal suffering, *and* we conquer the external behaviors that result from internal suffering.

From time to time, most of us become overwhelmed by negative thoughts such as judgments about ourselves or others, limiting beliefs, worries, and obsessions. If you can break down the negative thought, as it arises, into its elements, you will find that you can observe these individual elements without getting caught in them. Your negative tapes then lose much of their gripping power. They are experienced more as releases from the deep mind and less as sufferings of the surface mind. This is catharsis in the true sense of the original Greek, which literally means "cleaning out."

As this catharsis gains momentum, the forces that cause thought to be driven, unconscious, and fixated get worked through. You find that states of alert calm happen more frequently and last longer, simply because you have cleared out what gets in the way of this natural state. You are beginning to experience what the Bible refers to as "the peace that passeth understanding."

WHAT IS EQUANIMITY?

Equanimity is one of the most critical components you can develop as you begin to work with your pain. Equanimity is a fundamental skill for self-exploration and emotional intelligence. It is a deep and subtle concept, frequently misunderstood and easily confused with suppression of feeling, apathy, or inexpressiveness.

Equanimity comes from the Latin word aequus, meaning balanced, and animus, meaning spirit or internal state. As an initial step in understanding this concept, let's consider for a moment its opposite: what happens when a person loses internal balance.

In the physical world, we say a person has lost balance if they fall to one side or another. In the same way, a person loses internal balance if they fall into one or the other of the following contrasting reactions:

- Suppression: A thought and/or body sensation arises, and we attempt to cope with it by stuffing it down, denying it, tightening around it, and so on
- Identification: A thought and/or body sensation arises and we fixate on it, hold onto it inappropriately, not letting it arise, spread and pass with its natural rhythm

Between suppression on one side and identification on the other lies a third possibility, the balanced state: equanimity. There are two ways to develop equanimity.

One is to learn to intentionally create it, and the other is to recognize when you spontaneously fall into it.

Intentionally creating equanimity in your body is essentially equivalent to attempting to maintain a continuous relaxed state over your whole body as sensations (pleasant, unpleasant, strong, subtle, physical, emotional) wash through.

Intentionally creating equanimity in your mind means attempting to let go of negative judgments about what you are experiencing, and replacing them with an attitude of loving acceptance and gentle matter-of-factness. Notice my choice of words. I said, "Let go of negative judgments as they arise"; I did not say, "Try to get rid of them."

Let me give you a tangible example of how equanimity can be created in your body and mind. Let's say that you have a strong sensation in one part of your body. As you focus attention on what is happening over your whole body, you notice that you are tensing your jaw, clenching your fists, tightening your gut, and scrunching your shoulders. Each time you become aware of tensing in some area, you intentionally relax it to whatever degree possible. A moment later, you may notice that the tensing has started again in some area; once again, gently relax it to whatever degree possible. If there are areas that cannot be relaxed much or at all, you try to accept the tension sensations and just observe them.

As a result of maintaining this whole-body relaxed state, you may begin to notice subtle flavors of sensation spreading from the local area of intensity and coursing through your body. These are the sensations that you had been masking with tension. Now that they have been uncovered, try to create a mental attitude of welcoming them, not judging them. Observe them with gentle matter-of-factness, giving them permission to dance their dance, to flow as they wish through your body.

Even more important than creating equanimity is *recognizing when it occurs spontaneously*. Everyone, from time to time, falls into states of equanimity. If we are alert to this whenever it happens, and use it as an opportunity to explore the nature of equanimity, then it will happen more frequently and last longer.

For example, let's say that you have been working with a physical discomfort. At some point, you notice that, even though the discomfort level itself has not changed, it somehow seems to bother you less. Upon investigation, you realize that you have spontaneously fallen into a state of gentle matter-of-factness. By being alert to this, and by exploring the state, you are training your subconscious to produce the state more frequently.

Equanimity belies the adage that "you can't have your cake and eat it too." When you apply equanimity to unpleasant sensations, they flow more readily, and, as a result, cause less suffering. When you apply equanimity to pleasant sensations, they also flow more readily, and, as a result, deliver deeper fulfillment. The same skill positively affects both sides of the sensation picture. Hence the following equation:

Pain x Equanimity = Psychospiritual Purification = Pleasure x Equanimity

Furthermore, when feelings are experienced with equanimity, they assume their proper function as motivators and directors of behavior, as opposed to driving and distorting behavior. Thus, equanimity plays a critical role in changing negative behaviors such as substance and alcohol abuse, compulsive eating, violence, and so forth.

Equanimity is not at all the same as apathy. Equanimity involves non-interference with the natural flow of subjective sensation. Apathy implies indifference to the controllable outcome of objective events. Thus, although seemingly similar, equanimity and apathy are actually opposites. Equanimity frees up internal energy for effectively responding to external situations. By definition, equanimity involves radical permission to feel, and, as such, is the opposite of suppression. As far as external expression of feeling is concerned, internal equanimity gives one the freedom to externally express or not express, depending on what is appropriate to the situation.

CHAPTER
THREE

A New Perspective on Pain

FLAVORS OF PAIN

Now that I have given you a description of the meditation experience, and defined some of the key concepts, such as equanimity and the notion of "divide and conquer," let's look at how to apply this knowledge directly to working with pain.

Pain comes in various "flavors" or types: burning, aching, shooting, itching, pressure, and nausea are examples of flavors of pain. A person may experience several flavors simultaneously, and a given flavor may vary in its intensity. For example, an ache may range from mild to fainting intensity. What makes the method of "observing and opening" so extraordinary and powerful is that it works for all types of painful experience, regardless of the type of pain, its intensity, or its cause.

What exactly do I mean when I say "it works?" The benefits experienced by a person who uses this method come under two categories: First, it reduces the suffering caused by the specific pain you are dealing with. Second—and this is the really important point—working with your pain in this way fosters rapid personal evolution, a releasing of psychological and spiritual blockages, a kind of deep and permanent cleansing of the very substance of your soul. To borrow language from the Christian tradition, the experience of pain stops being "Hell" (that is to say, meaningless suffering), and turns into "Purgatory" (a purification that opens the way for direct encounter with the Spiritual Source). As a result of this purification, you will eventually experience an increased sense of oneness and connectedness with all things; a decrease in negative emotions such as anger, fear, sorrow, and guilt; a sense of happiness independent of your circumstances; and the disappearance of imprints and limiting conditioning from the past.

Associated with this transformation of consciousness is a distinct feeling, which I call the flavor of purification. It is the good feeling that comes as a person is experiencing painful feelings in a skillful way. Once you begin to develop a taste for this flavor of purification, pain (even horrible pain) becomes meaningful. Suffering diminishes and is eventually eclipsed by the joy of purification. This is what I mean by escaping into pain. If the pain is severe, and you are able to escape into it, you will experience an egoless state, a direct communion with the Spiritual Source.

The method of mindfulness applied to pain may appear to be very challenging. At first, you may not have good concentration. Your mind will wander a lot, and you will have to bring it back over and over again, but just as in any other exercise, skill comes with time and practice. So be patient with yourself, and although the mind may wander, keep returning to your meditation technique.

MINDFULNESS MEDITATION EXPERIENCE

What I would like to do now is take just a moment to give you a tangible sense of what I mean by mindfulness in relation to body sensation. Close your eyes and let your whole body relax and settle in. Pick one area where the pain is significant.

Get a clear sense of the size and shape of the painful region. Is it a long strip, round, triangular, or some other shape? Is it flat like a pancake, or does it have a three-dimensional volume? Is it uniform, or does it have areas of greater or lesser intensity within it? Are its borders sharp or diffuse? Does it spread any influence through the body, or is it completely isolated? You now have a much clearer and more precise sense of the painful sensation.

Now observe even more carefully, as though the pain were a living being in its own right—as though it were, for example, a lizard on a wall. How and when will this creature move? Will its borders change? Will it get stronger or weaker? Will its center shift? Watch very carefully for a while, and notice that, every few seconds, the pain may change, if only in a tiny way. Every time the pain changes in any little way, relax your whole mind and body into it, and just observe it without judgment.

Congratulations! You have taken your first step in developing the skill of mindfulness. It is true that sometimes the pain may seem to get worse as you focus on it. This, however, is a temporary phenomenon. If you can just stay with it, the suffering will often naturally break up after this temporary worsening.

HOW PAIN BECOMES SUFFERING

In order to understand how pain becomes suffering, you need to know a deep truth about the nature of suffering. Most people equate suffering with pain, but in fact, suffering is a function of two variables, not just one.

Once again, let me give you a metaphor: The area of a rectangle is a function of two variables—its height and its length. If you double the length, you double the area, although the height stays the same. If you reduce the height to zero, the area becomes zero no matter how long the original rectangle may have been.

In the same way, suffering is a function of two variables: pain, and the degree to which the pain is being resisted. What do I mean by resistance? Resistance occurs in both the body and the mind, and may be either conscious or unconscious. Conscious resistance in the mind takes the form of judgment, wishes, fearful projections, and so on: "I hate the pain. I can't stand this pain. When is it going to stop?" Conscious resistance in the body takes the form of tension and holding. You have pain in the leg, but you may be tightening the jaw, tensing the breath, perhaps clenching throughout the whole body, not letting the pain spread and circulate.

As for the unconscious resistance, by definition, we have no control over this, as it occurs in the deep preconscious level of neural processing, moment by moment. However, carefully observing the pain allows the unconscious to gradually unlearn its habit of resistance. This is why the practice of mindfulness often involves intently pouring awareness on the pain.

The formula "suffering equals pain multiplied by resistance" contains both good news and bad news. The good news is that, at least in theory, no one ever has to suffer, because resistance can be made very small, and eventually reduced to zero, through exercises such as those on the accompanying guided meditation CD. When the resistance factor becomes zero, suffering is zeroed out, no matter how big the pain factor may be.

What is the bad news? In many cases, resistance grows if the pain persists. Even though the pain may stay the same, the perceived suffering becomes unbearable because the resistance has become so large. Furthermore, according to this model, even tiny, subliminal pain can cause immense suffering if you strongly resist it. The suffering that underlies many forms of compulsive behavior, such as substance abuse, is often caused by subtle, subliminal pain that is subject to immense subconscious resistance. In working with pain, remember: subtle is significant!

ACCEPTANCE IS NOT INDIFFERENCE

At this point in our discussion, it would be good to address two areas of immense confusion: First, it is important to keep in mind that dropping resistance to the subjective flow of pain in no way implies that you stop resisting the objective source of the pain. In other words, accepting the pain in no way implies a passive surrender to the illness or hurtful circumstances causing the pain. In fact, as you get more and more skillful in opening to the pain, the energy that was being wasted in fighting with the pain is now freed up to fight for recovery and to live your life despite the pain. Although you do not and should not surrender to the objective situation of being ill, you try to surrender to the subjective sensations that the illness causes. This reduces your suffering and increases your energy.

The second point is that, although the suffering diminishes as resistance drops, the pain may stay, thus preserving the proper function of pain in nature as a warning, motivation, and so on. In other words, it is sometimes necessary to feel pain, but it is never necessary to suffer. Pain informs and motivates. Suffering drives and distorts. Pain experienced skillfully brings us closer to our Spiritual Source. Suffering alienates us from our Spiritual Source and our fellow human beings. Suffering obscures the perfection of the moment. Pain experienced skillfully *is* the perfection of the moment.

PAIN WITHOUT SUFFERING

For most people, the notion of pain that is not suffering may sound like an oxymoron, a contradiction in terms. Most people have difficulty imagining what the experience of pain without suffering would be like. Does it hurt? Yes. Is that a problem? No.

People have difficulty understanding this because they are not familiar with the experience of pure pain, that is, pain without resistance. Since much of our habitual resistance to the flow of pain begins at the preconscious level of neural processing, by the time we consciously experience a wave of pain, it has already been frozen into suffering by unconscious resistance. In other words, most of us cannot remember experiencing pure pain. What people call "pain" is actually a combination of pain and resistance.

I might add, parenthetically, that most people also are not familiar with the experience of pure pleasure. What people call "pleasure" is actually a mixture of pleasure and grasping around the pleasure. Just as consciousness is purified by experiencing pain without resistance, it is equally purified by experiencing pleasure without grasping. The dropping of resistance to pain and the letting go of grasping onto pleasure are two sides of equanimity.

I'd like to clarify a bit more what I mean by resistance. Your nervous system has built-in structures that produce and transmit pain signals. We might refer to them as pain circuits. They are part of you, just as your arms and legs are part of you. Left to themselves, they function spontaneously and effortlessly as part of the flow of Nature, like wind through the trees or ripples on a lake. They have one job and one job only: when stimulated, they produce a kind of energy wave that we humans call pain.

But as the result of a long conditioning process, human beings have also developed another part of ourselves: resistance. Resistance interferes with that energy wave, fights against it, tries to beat it back. Thus, deep within our being, there is a kind of violent conflict, a veritable civil war between two parts of the same system. This produces a pressure called suffering. The suffering will continue until either the pain circuits are no longer stimulated, or until the resistance drops away. Since suffering is produced by one part of you fighting with another part of you, there is obviously a deep link between the process of learning to experience pain without suffering, and the process of becoming more integrated and less self-conflicted.

According to this view, resistance is a kind of internal friction—the system grinding against itself. Now, consider the results of friction in a mechanical system, such as your car: If the car is not properly oiled, the pistons grind against the cylinders. This produces unwanted effects. It produces useless heat, wastes fuel, and may even warp the engine itself. In the same way, resistance to pain produces useless suffering, and wastes physical and psychological energy. Furthermore, the suffering may warp your perceptions and behavior.

The distortion in perception and behavior can be a big part of the horror of the pain. If the pain persists or is chronic, a person may begin to act out of character, and alienate friends, family, and caregivers. Fortunately, there are a number of effective ways to deal with this:

First, try to remember that it is the suffering that is making the world look so grim and causing you to act out of character. God (or Nature) never intends that we suffer, only that we sometimes feel pain. As you learn mindfulness and equanimity, these distorting effects drop away.

Second, be willing to forgive yourself and others, over and over again. You have been given a big homework assignment. The good news is that you do not have to turn it in right away. You are not expected to necessarily get it right the first time around. It does not matter if you stray from the path, as long as you always return.

Third, remember impermanence: The periods of distortion do not last forever. As the Bible says, "This, too, shall pass."

Fourth, you can create and use a support structure of individuals and organizations that can give you objective feedback and get you back on track when you become mired in subjective suffering. You will learn more about how to do this later on.

PAIN AND PURIFICATION

Many spiritual traditions around the world involve the practice of asceticism, which means spiritual purification through voluntarily taking on discomfort. The hair shirt and self-flagellation of Christian Europe, as well as the sweat lodges, sun dances, and vision quests of the American Indians, are examples of asceticism.

Perhaps the most spectacular spiritual practice of contemporary Native America is the Sun Dance, which began among the plains tribes, but in the last several decades has spread throughout the United States and Canada. The intensity and duration of sensations that are voluntarily accepted during that ceremony are almost beyond belief. The ceremony involves four days of dancing, sometimes in one-hundred-plus degree temperatures, with piercings skewered through the flesh, and with no food or liquid, and no mind-altering aids whatsoever.

You might doubt whether something like this is even physically possible, but every summer, several thousand Indian men, women, and children (as well as a smattering of non-Indians) take this on voluntarily and joyously. Unless you are a Native American, it is unlikely that you would have an opportunity to witness this extraordinary purification ceremony, although a version of it can be seen in the Richard Harris film, *A Man Called Horse.*

Another example of such practices, shown in a documentary during the Nagano Olympics, amazed television viewers around the world. The documentary was about the "marathon monks" of Mount Hiei, a monastery outside of Kyoto, the old capital of Japan. These monks practice what might be described as a spiritual ultra-marathon which, like the Sun Dance, would seem to be impossible and yet, like the Sun Dance, is taken on voluntarily and joyously in the interests of purifying oneself so that one may serve others. The monks take a vow to spend twelve years in isolation on that mountain. During that period, every winter for one hundred days in succession, they make a daily pilgrimage, beginning at the top of the mountain, going down to the base and into the city of Kyoto, and then back up to the top of the mountain. On the pilgrimage, they chant mantras and worship at every shrine and temple along the way, and indeed attempt to have spiritual communion with every tree and rock they encounter. The complete circuit takes about twenty hours, leaving only a few hours for sleep. Then they must begin again.

The monks must make this hundred-day pilgrimage each winter during their twelve years of isolation. In addition, twice during that twelve-year period, they must do a nine-day seated meditation, meaning that, for nine days, they sit without moving, without getting up, without sleeping, without eating, and without taking liquids.

When I lived in Japan, I had the privilege of personally meeting one of these marathon monks, staying at his temple, talking with him, and seeing how he spent his days. He told me that, before he transcended the pain, his legs sometimes hurt so much that he fantasized about having them cut off with a sword. When I first met him, I wondered to myself why anyone would put himself through such an excruciating ordeal.

As I stayed in his temple and observed his daily routine, the answer became evident. After going through twelve years of extreme ascetical practice, what does a person do with his days? The answer is simple: Having seen that which is beyond physical and emotional pain, he spent his days helping others do the same. People would come up from the city of Kyoto with this or that problem in their lives: a failed relationship, a runaway child, a drinking problem, depression, physical infirmities, and so forth. And he was simply there. They would talk to him, and by what he said and the place he was coming from as he said it, they would gain some solace and strength for their lives.

You might wonder what kinds of states a person passes through when sitting for nine days without eating, drinking, or moving. The monk I met told me that the first two days were very hard, but once he was past the second day, the rest was actually not so difficult because he found "the other side." You might think that the extremes of the Sun Dance or the marathon monks are irrelevant to people living in the contemporary world, but the fact is that, even with the best of curative and palliative medicine, you might well find yourself faced with intensity and duration of sensation comparable to what shamans and ascetics go through. For example, I remember that, when my father died of lung cancer, he hyperventilated constantly and did not eat or sleep for seven days as he slowly suffocated. Surely that is no less intense than anything that has been done voluntarily in the name of asceticism. My purpose in telling you these stories is to illustrate the fact that, even in the most extreme cases of intensity and duration of pain, it is possible not only to transcend, but to flourish.

Of course, if improperly understood, ascetical practice can become a form of egotism on one hand, or an expression of masochistic self-hatred on the other, but if properly understood, asceticism is a loving and gentle process of self-acceptance. Let me try to explain how this works: Just as pain multiplied by resistance equals suffering, pain multiplied by acceptance equals spiritual cleansing or purification. This tells us two important things: First, when pain is very intense, if you are able to maintain even a tiny degree of acceptance, then purification is still going on—that is, the pain is productive and meaningful. Second, even a small pain can bring significant purification if your attentiveness and equanimity are high. Thus, even though you may never do intense practices like the Christian renunciates or the Native American spiritual warriors, you may attain comparably deep purification. This can be achieved by bringing an extraordinary amount of openness to the ordinary aches and discomforts of daily life.

Furthermore, once you clearly understand that pain multiplied by equanimity equals purification, you are able to make a "conceptual reframing" of the pain. You are able to sacramentalize it—to see it as a kind of imposed monastery or sacred ceremony. Seeing pain as a natural monastery or imposed retreat for spiritual growth is particularly significant for those in chronic pain.

I have spoken of Mindfulness Meditation as being composed of two elements: an opening up to the pain, and a careful observing of the pain. The opening up fosters a process of spiritual purification. The careful observation leads to deep insight. This insight is like a many-sided jewel. Here, I will briefly discuss just one facet of this jewel, the aspect called impermanence.

INSIGHT INTO IMPERMANENCE

I sometimes ask students an odd sort of multiple-choice question: "Are the mountains moving?" The possible answers are "Yes," "No," and "It depends." I suggest that the correct answer is "It depends." It depends on how carefully and patiently you observe the mountains. Certainly, from the ordinary scale of time and space, a mountain seems very solid. Indeed, mountain is a metaphor for permanence. Yet, viewed microscopically, even mountains are a dance of energy. Vibrating molecules are made up of even more rapidly vibrating atoms, which are made up of even more rapidly vibrating elementary particles, and so forth.

Furthermore, viewed with the patience of centuries, as in a kind of super time-lapse photography, a mountain range would resemble the seething surface of the ocean or a rippling mass of protoplasm.

In the same way, your pain may seem as solid and permanent as a mountain, but as your powers of observation sharpen and your patience grows, you will probably begin to perceive aspects of change or impermanence. The sensation of pain shifts shape or position every few seconds, becomes stronger or weaker, expands, contracts, and circulates. Eventually, you come to realize that even the most horrible pain is, in fact, made up of vibrating atoms of pure energy. At this point, not only the pain, but the whole sense of a suffering self dissolves and becomes part of the flow of Nature, as effortless and refreshing as ripples spreading on a pond.

As insight into impermanence deepens, you come to realize that all seemingly solid experiences are, in fact, elastic, vibratory, porous, and transparent. With this realization, your understanding of yourself and the world goes through a remarkable and empowering shift in perspective. This is similar to some of the paradigm shifts of modern physics. Matter can also be viewed as energy, and solid particles can be seen as vibrating waves. Paralleling this, your material body can be experienced as a field of energy, and your sense of separate, solid self can dissolve into a wave. As a wave, you can experience oneness with all Creation. You become spiritual in the literal sense of the Latin word *spiritus*, which means "breath" or "wind"—something insubstantial, yet powerful.

IN SUMMARY

As soon as pain arises in the body, the mind becomes preoccupied with how to get relief. If you have understood my point, you now know that there are two kinds of relief, both of which are valid. There is temporary or conditional relief that comes through eliminating a particular pain, and there is permanent or unconditional relief that comes through retraining your relationship to any and all pain. If temporary relief is not possible, then become ardently preoccupied with the noble quest for permanent relief!

CHAPTER
FOUR

Practical Tips for Working with Pain

SO FAR, I HAVE presented you with a basic perspective on how to meditate with pain. That basic perspective could be summarized in one sentence: when observed with enough precision and patience, pain fosters spiritual insight and emotional purification. Now, I would like to cover a few specific areas where people often have questions, and then continue with a brief introduction to the five meditation techniques we will be working with.

BEGRUDGING DOWNTIME

People often resent the fact that the pain takes time away from life, preventing them from participating in the meaningful activities of work and play. And indeed, unless you understand how to use the situation to evolve and purify consciousness, time spent in pain is wasted and meaningless.

Fortunately, you can make a conceptual reframing that changes the meaning of time spent with pain. If Nature has given you so much pain that you cannot do anything else other than be with it, then there is a message here: you are not expected to be doing anything else! In other words, spending time—even long periods of time—just feeling pain is a legitimate calling in the eyes of God and Nature. Assuming that you are making at least some effort to purify and evolve consciousness by being with the pain in a skillful way, you are engaged in productive and meaningful work.

When you do any job, there is benefit both to yourself in the form of salary, and to others in the form of goods or services delivered. When you are assigned the job of being in pain, you receive payment in the form of transformation of your consciousness, and you perform an important service to others by becoming an example to them—a source of hope, inspiration, and empowerment. Your friends and family will all benefit from the "new and improved" you that results from this work.

Consider even the most extreme case: a person in so much pain that they can do nothing but lie in bed, seeing very few people, perhaps with no prospect of recovery, perhaps dying. You might think that in such an extreme case, even if the meditation were to help the victim, there would not be any broader benefit to humanity, but this may not necessarily be true.

Although the theory is quite controversial, a few scientists postulate the existence of morphogenic fields. This theory states that, whenever a person makes a breakthrough, it becomes easier for all others to have similar breakthroughs. This is sometimes referred to as the "hundredth monkey effect." According to this theory, a person isolated and cut off from contacts, who is working to purify themselves through pain, is, in some way, making it easier for all other sufferers in the world to do the same—a worthwhile and meaningful job indeed!

MELTING AND FREEZING

Next, I would like to discuss the phenomenon of "melting and freezing." Sometimes, as you are observing and opening to the pain, you may experience the pain softening. Sometimes, it softens just slightly, flowing like thick molasses or lava. Other times, it may become quite fluid and vibratory, expanding and contracting in an amoeba-like way, or even breaking up into a shower of champagne bubbles and subtle energy, like an atomizer sprayer. If that happens, enjoy it and concentrate on the vibrations and undulations, letting them relax you, massage you, and take you into a place of peace and safety.

After long and consistent practice of Mindfulness Meditation, such experiences of impermanence happen more frequently. However, it is of the utmost importance not to make this the goal of your meditation. The only goal is to do your best to carefully observe and open to the pain as it is. Whenever you do this, you are helping along a natural process of purifying and evolving yourself, whether or not you consciously experience any change in pain at that moment.

In the course of this purification, the pain may melt, but it may also freeze up again for various lengths of time. As a result of your meditation, the pain may actually get worse for a short period of time before you experience permanent transformation. When the pain melts, there is a tendency to think that the meditation is working, that you are making progress, or that you are doing it right, but if the pain "refreezes," you may think the meditation is not working, or that you are doing it wrong. Always remember the definition of a successful meditation session: a successful meditation is any meditation you did!

Consciousness is a many-layered structure. Like the geological strata of the earth, the deeper layers contain older fossils. As you are pouring clarity and openness on your pain, the pain is actually functioning as a conduit or tunnel into the deepest reaches of your subconscious mind. As a layer of psychological blockage comes to the surface, it may cause the pain to solidify or get worse. Just open to that, and keep on observing as much as possible, without an agenda that the pain soften or go away. It is part of Nature's wry sense of humor that the quickest way to "break up" pain is to observe it without the slightest desire that it be different in any way.

So, if the pain melts and then gets hard and harsh once again, remember: you have not gone backwards, but rather a deeper level of blockage has percolated upwards. You may go through many cycles of softening and re-congealing. The English poet T.S. Eliot, who was also a Christian mystic, vividly describes this aspect of the spiritual path in his Four Quartets. He writes, "Between melting and freezing, the soul's sap quivers."

WHEN AND WHERE TO MEDITATE

People sometimes ask me, "How many hours a day do you meditate?" They are, of course, referring to the amount of time I spend in formal sitting practice. I answer, "Usually about an hour a day," but often I feel like saying, "I meditate twenty-four hours a day, hopefully." In other words, meditation can be carried on during the daily activities of life, as well as during set formal periods. Both forms of practice are useful. If your focus of meditation is pain, then you can be meditating any time you feel the pain, because whenever you are observing and opening to it, you are, by definition, meditating. If pain is always present, then you have a reminder and motivation to be in a meditative state all your waking hours, like the monks and nuns in monastic training. In this sense, pain can become an ally.

Of course, it takes practice to meditate on pain while at the same time engaging in other activities. At first, it will be challenging enough to meditate quietly by yourself, but as the state of concentration becomes habitual, you will be able to meditate in the midst of life activities.

Try to set aside a period of time most days for formal meditation—perhaps a half an hour each morning. Of course, if your pain prevents you from doing other activities, you may be formally meditating for many hours each day. You can meditate sitting in a chair or on the floor, or lying down. During your periods of formal meditation, make sure that there will be no distractions. Turn off the phones. Let friends and family know that you need to be alone for a short period of time.

Meditation is a state of both relaxation and alertness. If you meditate in a seated posture, try to keep the spine straight. This will help you to remain alert. If you meditate lying down, you must have very strong determination not to let your mind sink into sleepiness or even fuzziness. If you become even slightly drowsy, open your eyes with an unfocused gaze, as if staring at infinity, without fixing your gaze on visual objects. This will help you remain aware and alert.

The most important moment in any period of formal meditation comes when you get up to resume your daily activities. Your ability to maintain a meditative state throughout the day (and hence reduce the suffering from your pain) depends on how you handle this transition. Instead of thinking, "The meditation is over, now it's time to do this or that," think, "I have become somewhat more calm and focused. Now my job is to try to preserve this state."

Make the transition gradually. After a period of meditating, either with the CD or on your own, slowly stand in place for a few minutes, and try to maintain a focused state as you stand. Then walk around the room, and see if you can preserve that state while walking. Then go do some simple task that does not require thinking, like washing the dishes. Try to do that task within a meditative state. Finally, move on to the complex activities of your day. Whenever you become agitated or start to suffer a lot from pain during the day, drop everything for a few minutes. Sit or lie down and do a short, but high-quality "mini-meditation" to re-ground yourself. Do this as many times as needed throughout the day.

The combination of setting aside at least a half-hour each day for formal meditation and doing frequent mini-meditations will eventually allow you to maintain a state of deep calm and high focus for much, if not most, of your day.

FAINTING

When pain is extreme, you may feel like you are going to faint. Lie down and open up to that experience. Try to maintain your meditation technique through the fainting. With time, you will be able to maintain alertness and equanimity throughout the entire experience. Fainting now becomes an experience of deep meditation. You will feel that you have gone beyond the body and transcended suffering.

Admittedly, the notion of "mindfully fainting" may seem strange and frightening. It will probably take some practice before you can really "let go" into the faint. Eventually, you will come to learn that there is nothing whatsoever to fear in this situation, as long as you keep a level of mindfulness and openness.

SECONDARY SENSATIONS

Now I would like to briefly mention a phenomenon that I call "secondary sensations." In addition to the primary sensation of pain, you may have other sensations such as heat, nausea, fatigue, agitation, heebie-jeebies, jerking, creepy-crawly feelings, and so on. You may feel like your marrow is itching everywhere, bugs are crawling in your veins, or you are going to jump out of your skin. You may have pressures or tensions over your whole body.

Treat these secondary sensations in the same way you treat the pain itself. Observe them carefully and open up to them. Indeed, honor and welcome them, because they are an important part of the purification process. They often represent body memories percolating up from your pool of undigested past experiences. Your present physical pain is activating your body's subtle memory of past pains, both physical and emotional. These will magnify your sense of suffering from the present pain, unless you are able to clearly detect them and open up to them.

All you have to do is observe and open up to such secondary sensations the same way you observe and open up to the primary pain. This creates an optimal environment within which your unconscious can unburden itself. For years, unbeknownst to you, these subtle body memories have been continuously present in your unconsciousness, distorting every moment of your experience. By "feeling it through" now, you will find that each moment of your life to come will be easier and more fulfilling.

DEALING WITH EMOTIONS

Typically, physical pain produces emotional reactions, which may be quite intense. The most common emotional reactions can be grouped into four categories: The first is the fear family, which can range from subtle anxiety to paralytic terror. The second is the anger family, which can range from mild irritation to homicidal rage. The third is the sadness family, which can range from being slightly "down" to deep depression, and includes grieving and self-pity. The fourth family is the shame family, which can range from slight self-consciousness to intense humiliation or mortifying shame.

The same principles of mindfulness that work with physical pain can also be applied to such emotions. The important thing to remember is that emotions consist of a combination of ideas in the mind and feelings in the body. Using the principle of divide and conquer, the ideas can be broken up into mental image and internal conversation, and the feelings can be broken up into flavors and locations. Then these components can be worked with individually until they begin to flow and dissolve.

CHAPTER
FIVE

Introduction to the Guided Meditations

ONE OF THE CHALLENGING aspects of working with pain is a kind of built-in "Catch-22": Until you have actually experienced the resistance breaking up and pain turning into waves and vibrations, it is difficult to believe that such a thing is even possible. On the other hand, unless you believe that such a thing is possible, it is difficult to keep meditating on the pain long enough for this to happen. It is sometimes necessary to meditate continuously on the pain for many hours before the resistance begins to soften.

This is where the guided meditations come in. I present three basic strategies for working with your pain: focusing on the pain, focusing on your mental and emotional reactions to the pain, or focusing away from the pain onto something soothing and pleasant.

Track Two gives you a procedure for monitoring your reactions to the pain. Tracks Three and Four offer guidance for focusing on the discomfort itself. Track Five offers guidance for focusing away from the discomfort. Each of these approaches has payoffs and challenges associated with it. I would encourage you to alternate the three methods, because at any given time, one method may be more effective than another. These practices are designed so that you can either listen to them straight through, or listen for awhile, turn them off, meditate on your own, and then resume listening. In this way, through switching back and forth between working with the guided practices and working on your own, you can build the critical mass of continuous concentration needed to take the suffering out of the pain.

By sometimes working under audio guidance and sometimes working on the procedure on your own, you will eventually internalize these skills, so you will need to rely less and less on the CD. On the other hand, even after you have internalized these techniques, you can always return to the CD for support when you face a strong challenge.

TRACK ONE

How to Use This CD

Here, I reiterate the general principles of working with your pain in conjunction with the guided meditations that follow. Listen to this track before you begin the meditations for the first time, and return to it whenever you feel a need to review the basic concepts or re-motivate yourself to practice.

TRACK TWO

Emotional Reactions to Pain

When I work one-on-one with people in pain, I usually have them start by tracking their subjective reactions to the pain. In terms of tangible sensory experience, what do we mean by a subjective reaction to pain? At any given instant, the physical discomfort in the body may trigger a mental comment, that is to say, internal talk. For example, you might find yourself constantly drawn to phrases like, "This is horrible … What am I going to do? … What if it gets worse? … Why me? … I've got to do something about this pain …" and so forth. However, it is also possible, in a specific instant, that there might be no internal talk triggered by the discomfort. In other words, verbal thinking could either be stimulated by the discomfort, or it could be quieted by the discomfort.

At any given instant, the physical discomfort might trigger a mental picture. For example, you might see an image of the place in the body where the discomfort is, or an image of the energy of the discomfort, or an archetype that represents the discomfort, such as a hammer pounding you or a knife cutting you.

It is also possible that the discomfort might turn off mental pictures, causing your mental screen to fill either with light or darkness that washes away the images.

Finally, at any given instant, the physical discomfort may cause an emotional feeling in the body. By emotional feeling, I mean body sensations such as anger, fear, sadness, impatience, and so forth.

The most typical feeling triggered by physical discomfort is, of course fear, but teariness or sadness, anger, and impatience are not uncommon. It is also possible that the physical discomfort could trigger pleasant emotions, such as interest, or even gratitude. So once again, at any given instant, the physical discomfort might cause an emotional feeling in the body.

On the other hand, sometimes the physical sensation of the discomfort is so great that it turns off all emotional feeling, putting you in a very impersonal state. This is not necessarily bad. The turning off of emotional feeling could be interpreted as a kind of emotional rest, just as the quiet is rest from verbal thought, and the clear light or deep darkness is rest from visual thought.

So, taken together, at any given instant, one's reaction to the discomfort must fall exactly into one of the following eight possibilities:

1. Feeling (body sensations of anger, fear, sadness, impatience, and so on)
2. Imagery (mental pictures, visual thought)
3. Talk (self-talk, mental comments)
4. Imagery and Feeling (two modalities at the same time)
5. Talk and Feeling (another case of two modalities at the same time)
6. Imagery and Talk (yet another case of two modalities at the same time)
7. Feeling and Imagery and Talk (all three modalities at the same time)
8. None (thought and feeling reactions have ceased; you are resting in the state of no self)

There are several payoffs to working with feeling/image/talk reactions to physical discomfort. For one thing, you may become overwhelmed at some point, and want to give up on meditating. If, at the very instant this occurs, you pay close attention to what is going on, you will discover that the desire to give up is nothing more than a sudden and intense eruption of feel/image/talk. If you know how to track these elements, you will not be ambushed by that reaction. In other words, you will not automatically buy into the feel/image/talk, and give up. Rather, you will be able to see your desire for what it is. Thus, by knowing how to track your reactions, you will be able to continue the meditative process in spite of urges to stop. That is one payoff.

A second payoff has to do with the reduction of your suffering. Some of the interference with the natural flow of pain comes about because of the feel/image/talk reactions to the pain. Therefore, by working with those feel/image/talk reactions, you will reduce some of the resistance to the pain. Since suffering equals pain multiplied by resistance, this will result in a reduction of suffering. However, there is a subtle point to be considered: You are not trying to get rid of the feel/image/talk reactions. That is impossible, although they may stop on their own. What you are trying to do is to let them come and go without identifying with them. It is not the presence of these reactions, but rather the fact that we lock onto them, that causes them to turn into resistance that then multiplies with the discomfort, vastly increasing our sense of suffering.

Therefore, you have to actually welcome the feel/image/talk reactions, and let them play themselves out in a natural way. So, a second benefit is that, by working with the feel/image/talk reactions, you will reduce "cross-multiplication," and therefore reduce your suffering.

Another benefit of working with the categories of feel/image/talk is that you can not only notice when you have reactions, but you can also know what to look for so that you can spot the absence of reactions. I said that Nature does not intend us to suffer. In other words, the pain itself contains the answer to pain. When the pain becomes very intense, we say, "It hurts so much I can't think straight … It hurts so much I can't see straight … It hurts so much I feel depersonalized."

In point of fact, that is simply the pain turning off the feel/image/talk reactions to itself. Instead of seeing that as a problem, you can experience the pain taking you into a state of pure light or pure darkness, deep quiet and transpersonal self. In that case, even if the pain itself remains very intense, you will experience a state of freedom from the feel/image/talk self, which could be called no self or the transpersonal self. No self, no problem!

There are many specific procedures for monitoring or observing feel/image/talk reactions. Track Two of this CD represents just one of these procedures, which I have found comes quite naturally for most people.

TRACK THREE
Free-Floating within the Discomfort
This track is the first of two meditations designed to help you focus on the discomfort itself. The advantage of focusing on the discomfort is that it will allow you to bring equanimity to the discomfort. This reduces suffering, and will eventually allow you to experience discomfort as a flow of energy. Ultimately, the desperation of suffering is transformed into the taste of purification.

Track Three is designed to give you the general picture of your discomfort by having you free-float within it. It is also designed to sensitize you to when the discomfort begins to break up into energy by having you notice, second by second, whether the discomfort is stable or changing. At any given instant, the discomfort that you are focusing on will either be perfectly stable, or it will be changing in some way, perhaps subtly, in intensity, in quality, or in shape.

Our goal is never to get the sensations to change, but simply to be sensitive to the fact that they may change. If they do change, become fascinated with the change. The more fascinated you become with the change, the more you drop into equanimity; the more you drop into equanimity, the less you will resist the flow of the pain, and so the pain becomes more flowing. By creating this positive feedback loop, we are aiding the natural process of the dissolution of the pain.

TRACK FOUR
Working With Local Intensity and Global Spread
On Track Four, we deal with the interplay of local intensity and spread. When you have physical discomfort in your body, that discomfort may assume one of several spatial configurations: Very commonly, there will be one area, or several disconnected areas of noticeable intensity. In addition to those areas of intensity, there may be areas of lesser intensity caused by the spread of sensation from the local areas. The spread of the discomfort may fill part of the body, or the whole body, or even seem to go beyond the borders of the body in one or more directions.

Another possibility is that there are no local areas of intensity, but instead, the entire body is inundated with more or less uniform discomfort. In a sense, the entire body is one local sensation. Yet another possibility is that there are one or more areas of local intensity, and no spread at all.

If spread is present, it can be a very productive object to focus on. Often, the bulk of your suffering is not actually in the local intensities, but in the tightening around the subtle spread from those local intensities. This track gives you a process for working with that spread, as well as with the local intensities themselves.

I mentioned that, when I work one-on-one with people in pain, I often start by having them track their feel/image/talk reactions. After that, the next thing I have people do is to see if there is any spread, and if so, I have them work with that spread for a while. There are two reasons for doing this: First, as I mentioned, a lot of suffering results from subliminal freezing around that spread. Second, because the spread is usually much weaker than the local intensity, it may be possible to have a high degree of equanimity with the spread, even though it may not be possible to completely accept the local intensities. Therefore, working with spread, when it is present, represents a skillful means. One can use the fact that the spread is less horrible than the local intensities to cultivate a high degree of equanimity with it. This allows the spread to flow, and that, in turn, creates a space into which the pressure from local intensity can dissipate. So, my strategy is to first look into talk/image/feel reactions, then investigate the possibility of spread, and finally focus on the primary pain, which by this point may be noticeably less intense.

TRACK FIVE
Breath Pleasure

In addition to focusing on one's feel/image/talk reactions and focusing on the discomfort itself, you also have the option of attempting to focus away from the discomfort but there is a subtle point here that you must keep in mind: meditatively focusing away from discomfort is not the same as distracting yourself from the discomfort. Distracting yourself is certainly an acceptable coping strategy for pain, but it is not a source of strength and growth. Distraction is, in a sense, a form of anesthetic, a palliative that brings temporary relief.

Meditatively focusing away from the discomfort is a completely different process; it is the process of developing your concentration skills by repeatedly pulling attention away from the discomfort and focusing it on some other object. The difference between distraction and focusing away lies in the intention. I am not suggesting that you should not distract yourself, if you find that it is helpful. I am only saying that meditatively focusing away is a different process, one that requires work, but has growth potential.

Let me give you a metaphor: When you lift a weight, you work against the force of gravity, and by doing that work, muscle is built. In the same way, by intentionally pulling yourself away from the pain, and continuously focusing on something else, you are working against the gravitational pull of the pain. In this way, your concentration muscle is built.

As I have repeatedly emphasized, concentration is a generic skill. After you have practiced developing it with one object of experience, you can apply it to any object of experience. So, paradoxically, the concentration power that you develop by meditatively focusing away from the pain can later on be used to focus on the pain, or on your reactions to the pain.

Furthermore, focusing away from the pain and onto something that is soothing may create a state of equanimity within you.

You could focus away from the pain onto music; you could even focus on television or a conversation. However, one natural object to focus on is your breath, assuming that there is not a lot of pain in the breath itself. There are a number of reasons why you might choose the breath as the object of your focus: First, it is always there, whereas music or television may not be. Second, there is a link between the breathing process and the pain process, so that, if you focus on the breath in the way described in this integrated book/CD, it will tend to free up the breathing process, which can actually help relieve the pain. In hospitals, oxygen is often given to people for pain. Working meditatively with your breath can bring about similar effects.

The technique on Track Five involves contacting two flavors of pleasure within the breath: one is the pleasure of relaxing as you breathe out, and the other is the pleasure of oxygen intake as you breathe in. You will probably be able to detect at least one of these. If you find the out-breath productive, you can focus just on the pleasure of relaxing as you breathe out. If you find that the in-breath productive, you can focus just on the pleasure of oxygen intake as you breathe in. If both seem productive, you can alternate between the two.

Finding pleasure within the breath is significant in working with pain, because pain tends to disrupt the breathing process. By finding pleasure within the breath, you are breaking up some of that interference.

As you begin to relax, there are several ways in which relaxation may affect your experience of the pain: One possibility is that it will have no particular effect on the pain. A second possibility is that it will reduce the suffering due to pain, because you are entering a state of equanimity and you are tightening less around the pain.

However, a third possibility is that relaxation can make the pain seem worse, at least temporarily. If this occurs, it is important to know two things: why it is happening, and what to do about it.

So, why would relaxing make the pain seem worse? Because we cope with pain though all sorts of tensions in the body, and as we remove those tensions, the pain can spread, because you are not holding it in with tension anymore. What to do? To the best of your ability, give the pain permission to spread.

TRACK SIX
Winding Up
As you finish a period of meditation, it is important to return to your life smoothly and slowly, without losing the meditative state you have achieved. As you return to a standing position, focus on the qualities of concentration, equanimity, restfulness, or energy flow that may have developed. Sometimes pain may intensify as you begin activities, so it is important to keep your meditative tools in place throughout the transition process. Do not be discouraged if pain remains after your initial meditation sessions. These procedures often require repeated practice.

STICKING WITH YOUR PRACTICE
I would strongly encourage you to continue the meditation session until there has been at least some reduction in suffering. If the discomfort is deep or intense, that may take several hours. Although this prospect might seem daunting, the fact is that

the pain is going to be there anyway, whether you work with it intentionally or not, so why not work with it? Certainly, that is preferable to abject suffering.

When you do achieve some relief—either because of dropping into equanimity, or because the pain itself breaks up into energy—you will have learned something that completely changes your perspective on life. The more times you accomplish this, the easier it becomes. You become intimately familiar with each step in the process. Pain is part of Nature, but hours and hours of suffering are not what Nature intends. In other words, there is a natural process whereby the body knows how to dissolve the very pain it produces. Unfortunately, human beings, by and large, are not familiar with that process, so they cannot help it along. In fact, they usually interfere with that process and, as a result, the suffering goes on and on and on, contrary to the principles of Nature.

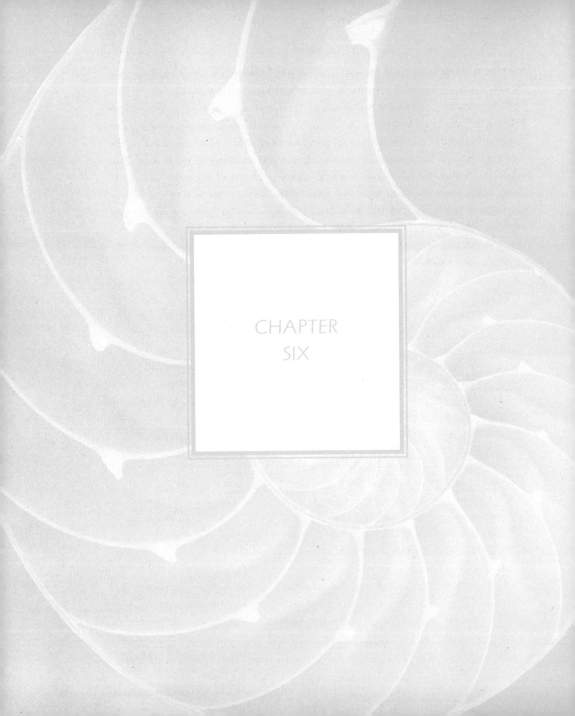

CHAPTER
SIX

Pain Relief in Action

OVER THE YEARS, I have worked with many people in physical discomfort, using the principles and techniques I have presented in this book. Some have come to me with acute pain issues, others with long-term chronic pain. I would like to share a few of their stories with you, so you can see how the pain relief process works in specific cases. As you will see in these stories, when a person is able to experience physical and emotional discomfort as a purification, it often leads quite naturally to a sense of love and compassion for others.

I would like to start with the story of a man I will call "Gene." He was the first person I guided through the dying process.

Gene was one of the toughest guys I ever met. He had been a sea captain during WWII, and had twice survived having his ship blown up. He was a very colorful person, short and stocky, a chain smoker. I used to think of him as the living embodiment of Popeye the Sailor Man.

At the time we first met, I was the vice abbot and meditation instructor at the International Buddhist Meditation Center in Los Angeles. I had recently returned from Asia, and was still living very much as a monk. One day, when I was out doing work in the yard, Gene approached me. He explained to me that he had just punched out the head monk of a neighboring temple where he had been living. Of course, the temple had kicked him out, so he wanted to know if he could move into my center.

Now, as I mentioned before, I am basically pretty wimpy, and I could not help wondering when he might punch me out, too, but something in me said to give the guy a chance, so I allowed him to move in.

As you can imagine, Gene had a lot of unresolved life issues. He was already an older guy at this point. He was estranged from his family, and his own kids hated him. In a way, it was amazing that someone like him would even be attracted to meditation practice, but despite or because of all those issues, he took to meditation practice with great fervor.

One of the reasons I could relate to him was that I had studied under a great Taiwanese master named Wuguang. Before coming to Buddhist practice, Wuguang had been a really tough sailor in the Japanese merchant marine, with a reputation for pugnacity that was known all along the South China coast. I thought that, if Wuguang could become such a gentle and enlightened being, there was hope for Gene, too.

Eventually Gene moved away, but he continued his practice. About five years down the line, I got a call. "This is Gene," he said. "They say I have lung cancer and will die for sure in the next couple of months. Would you please come out and guide me through the process?"

I had never guided a person through the dying process, but I knew the basic principles, based on my own experience with dealing with various physical and emotional issues, and based on Buddhist writings, so I had a degree of confidence that I could help him. I agreed to go to Tulsa, Oklahoma, where he was then living, and work with him.

Over the course of several days, it became clear that he had five different kinds of discomfort in his body, five physical sensations he was dealing with. First, there was pain from the tumors themselves. Second, there was discomfort due to exhaustion. Third, he had nausea. Fourth, he had a degree of fear related to dying. Finally, as you might expect of someone with his history, he had a degree of irritability.

I had him work individually with each of those five body qualities. He began to tease out the differences between them: "the tumor pain feels this way, the exhaustion discomfort feels this way, and the nausea discomfort feels this way." He came to understand that they were really distinct sensory events.

I sat with him and guided him in techniques that allowed him to isolate the various flavors in his body, then explore how those flavors interacted with each other, then, once again, tease out the individual flavors—analysis, synthesis, analysis, synthesis, not once or twice, but over and over and over.

None of the pains went away. However, the sense of problem, the sense of overwhelm vastly diminished. Why did it diminish? Because when those qualities would occur together, he now experienced them as merely adding to each other, rather than cross-multiplying. Let's say that a person dying of cancer has ten units of exhaustion, ten units of tumor discomfort, ten units of nausea discomfort, ten units of anger discomfort and ten units of fear discomfort. By what mathematical formula do we compute their total suffering? Under ordinary circumstances, because the sensations reinforce each other, the formula would be something like ten times ten times ten times ten times ten, which equals one hundred thousand. No wonder people say, "Please let me die, I can't stand another moment ..." If they had perfect mindfulness skills, they would not say that. Their total experience of suffering would be exactly what is there: ten plus ten plus ten plus ten plus ten, which adds up to fifty.

If you think of the difference between having a fifty-pound weight on you and a one hundred thousand-pound weight on you, you will begin to get a sense of how awesome it is to divide and conquer. Because each of these sensations was clear and distinct, and because Gene had worked hard for five years with his meditation practice, he was readily able to "deconstruct" his suffering. Not only did it vastly reduce the suffering, but it allowed him to experience his illness and his death as a psychospiritual purification.

The ancient Greeks held that a good death was one of the goals of human life. By good death, they meant passing away without physical or emotional suffering. Indeed, they had a word for it—*euthanasia*. *Thanatos* means death; *thanasia* means the dying process, and *eu* means good. So, originally, *euthanasia* did not mean "mercy killing;" it meant "a good dying process." But the best dying occurs when one begins to experience the "taste of purification," which I described in Chapter Three. That is what happened to Gene.

Gene started to get the sense that, when the discomforts would occur, he was cleaning out the storehouse of his past actions. He would be vomiting in the bathroom, come out, and say something like, "Boy, I really let go of a lot of stuff with my son just then."

In the midst of working with Gene, I received a call from a friend in California who had just been diagnosed with a large tumor. My friend was understandably in shock and upset at the news he had just received. After speaking with him for a while, I put Gene on the phone. To this day, I am deeply moved when I recall that scene: Gene would say words of comfort and encouragement to my friend, then have a bout of violent vomiting, then go right back to comforting and encouraging my friend, then vomit again. Because Gene was experiencing his own discomfort with mindfulness and equanimity, it was purifying his consciousness, awakening in him a natural compassion for others.

Well, Gene did not die on schedule, and eventually I had to leave because of other commitments. He asked me for some parting advice, and I said, "Just keep separating those sense elements out and working with them. That's the most important advice I can give you now."

I can give you a metaphor for what this divide and conquer process feels like: You may have seen very skilled drummers that have four-limbed independence. You watch them, and your jaw drops. How can each limb be doing something entirely different? How can four limbs operate without interfering with each other? There is a certain way that the motor nerves for each limb are functioning so that they are not getting in each other's way, and it produces this incredibly graceful, clean, refreshing quality when you watch it. Each circuit is doing its job without interfering with the others.

Mindfulness Meditation creates the same kind of independence in one's sensory circuits. Each sensory system does its job without interfering with the others. This produces the subjective analog of that grace and refreshing clean quality. Even if you have many different kinds of physical and emotional sensations going on in your body, if they ripple through each other, interpenetrating without interfering, it is beautiful and refreshing, like the effect of rain drops on a pool of water.

The other story I would like to share is that of a woman named Shirley. Shirley's story is a case study in the effects of meditation on long-term pain. Early in life, Shirley was a gorgeous, healthy, and athletic woman. She was also very successful in business, working as a high-end corporate trainer and psychotherapist. Intelligent and brimming with people skills, she basically had it made.

Then she began to develop serious health issues. Although she heroically raised three wonderful children on her own and attempted to continue her career, she suffered through a seemingly endless series of health catastrophes and surgeries. She had multiple neurosurgeries to remove bone spurs from her spine and other parts of her body; she developed bowel cancer, and the subsequent operation then led to infection; she went through disc fusions and bone grafts in an attempt to repair the damage to her spine. In one bone graft, she was given some improperly irradiated foreign bone, which caused her immune system to shut down, so on top of everything else, she developed Chronic Fatigue Syndrome. All told, over a period of twenty years, she endured more than twenty major surgeries.

Shirley ended up not merely in chronic pain, but in chronic extreme pain—white-knuckle pain, every hour of the day. Eventually, the doctors simply could not operate any more, because the adhesions and scarring from the surgeries had become as damaging as the condition itself.

With this kind of pain, there is often a high probability that people will take their own lives. I suspect that that we are hardwired to move in this direction if there is nothing but pain day after day. The horrible part of chronic pain is that, the more it hurts, the more sensitive you become to the pain. Your pain circuits become pain magnifiers, so that even ordinary sensations are experienced as painful.

She explored every possible avenue for dealing with her pain—alternative medicine, healers, homeopathic remedies, therapies of various sorts. In 1974, she participated in the first hospital-based pain management program ever. But she was constantly having her hopes built up, and then shattered.

Shirley was always a spiritual seeker, and had investigated various spiritual teachers in the Los Angeles area. A friend of hers suggested that she might relate to my way of teaching. One Sunday, she came up and she introduced herself, and described her life. Initially, she did not actually come to me for meditation; she wanted my opinion on the ethics of taking her own life. She wondered whether it was justified for somebody in her situation to commit suicide. And I said, "I don't know the answer to that, but before you do something that radical, would you be willing to try something else?" That something else was Mindfulness Meditation.

I guess we are always attracted to challenges, and I looked upon Shirley's situation as a kind of "test case." If mindfulness practice could bring hope back to her life, it could do so in anyone's life. So I began to instruct her. It took countless hours of personal coaching over a period of many years, but in the end the results were nothing short of miraculous. Over those years, the pain actually got worse; however, her ability to transcend eventually outstripped the increasing pain.

When we first began working together, Shirley was using heavy medication for pain relief. She actually had a pump implanted in her body that delivered morphine directly to her spine. However, several years ago, the pump malfunctioned, and she went into a convulsive coma.

She was in the coma for several weeks, and the doctors wanted to pull the plug; they believed that she had suffered too much brain damage to survive on her own. However, Shirley's daughter, who is, herself, a doctor, refused to let that happen.

I spoke with the daughter about what might be happening to Shirley as she lay in coma. "You know," I said, "your mom has many years of meditation work, and something fundamental changes in the circuitry of the nervous system of someone who has practiced that long. Her brain circuits may be random right now, but that's not necessarily a bad thing." I believed that, if she did come out of the coma, there might actually be a number of positive effects, because neurological reorganization might have taken place. I certainly was not claiming with conviction that this would be the case, but in fact, that is exactly what happened.

Shirley came out of the coma, and within a few days, she was psychologically and spiritually clearer than ever. She soon made the decision to go off all medications, and to move from Los Angeles to San Francisco to be closer to her three grandchildren.

Now she now spends a great deal of time taking care of her grandchildren, which is certainly not something that most people in chronic pain are able to do. She also works as a volunteer at the Buddhist hospice in San Francisco, a job that even healthy people would find physically and psychologically challenging. She has found her calling in that work.

As a result of mindfulness practice, Shirley now lives a life of joyous and meaningful service, both as a committed hospice volunteer, and as a care provider for her grandchildren. This exemplifies the complete spiritual path—to transcend your own suffering, and then reach out to others in wisdom and compassion.

CHAPTER
SEVEN

Going Further

IN CONCLUSION, I want to thank you for being the kind of person who is ready to work with pain in the meditative way. At this point in human history, relatively few people are clear and courageous enough to take on this challenge. I also want to thank you for giving me the opportunity to share some of the things that I have learned over the last three decades. This sharing is my greatest source of joy. I wish you success in this noble quest.

You are not alone in your efforts to transcend pain and deepen your spiritual life. Meditation retreats, classes, and weekly sitting groups are available in most cities, and teachers in the mindfulness tradition may visit areas near you. Contact with teachers and other meditators will encourage and inform your practice. Participating in retreats and sitting groups allows you to build up a momentum of practice, so that, eventually, you can "break through" even horrible pain. As a next step after using this integrated book/CD, I strongly encourage you to investigate programs in your area, and participate in weekly group meditations and one-day, weekend, or longer retreats, if your life situation allows for this. I, myself, conduct retreats throughout North America. My teaching activities are coordinated through Vipassana Support International (VSI).

PERSONALIZED PAIN RELIEF GUIDANCE OVER THE PHONE OR THE INTERNET

One of the challenges in working with pain is that there are many individual variations in experience. Moreover, a given individual's experience may change rapidly moment by moment.

The methods of working with pain that are contained in this integrated book/CD represent the essence of my approach. However, in order to deal with the subtleties of individual variation and moment-by-moment change, you may wish to make use of my full, interactive Manage-Pain-Online system.

Using the Manage-Pain-Online system is remarkably close to having a personal session with me. Through this automated system I literally talk to you, you talk back, and based on your reports, the guidance changes, just as it would if we were working in person. The expert system logic contained within this program actually remembers your previous sessions and changes the guidance accordingly, thus assuring a unique and optimal experience each time you use it

Using this system is, in many ways, similar to using this integrated book/CD, but with more procedures and pathways. This leads to greater flexibility and greater potential to capitalize on natural windows of opportunity as they present themselves moment to moment.

Through this revolutionary new system, it is now possible to deliver personalized, high-quality coaching in mindfulness practice for hours on end, anywhere in the world, at any time. This is exciting because, as I have pointed out, it may take many hours of subtle guidance for a person to break through significant pain. An automated system can provide those hours of quality time on demand. As far as I know, this is the first time that artificial intelligence expert system technology has been used to facilitate meditative consciousness.

MANAGE PAIN ONLINE

To experience my interactive guided meditation program, visit: www.Manage-Pain-Online.com or call 800-456-8012.

VIPASSANA SUPPORT INTERNATIONAL

For articles covering a wide range of topics related to meditation and spiritual practice, as well as a schedule of my retreats for the year, visit the VSI website at: www.shinzen.org. To find out about meditation programs in your area, or to get help in establishing a meditation practice, contact Choshin Vamplew at VSI by calling toll free at 866-666-0874, or emailing vsi@shinzen.org.

About the Author

SHINZEN YOUNG became fascinated with Asian culture while a teenager in Los Angeles. Later he enrolled in the Ph.D. program in Buddhist Studies at the University of Wisconsin.

Eventually, he went to Asia and did extensive training in each of the three major Buddhist meditative traditions: Vajrayana, Zen, and Vipassana.

Upon returning to the United States, his intellectual interests shifted to the burgeoning dialogue between Eastern internal science and Western technological science. In recognition of his original contributions to that dialogue, the Institute of Transpersonal Psychology has awarded him an honorary doctorate.

Shinzen's innovative techniques for pain management derived from two sources: The first is his personal experience dealing with discomfort during intense periods of meditation in Asia, and during shamanic ceremonies with tribal cultures. The second is some three decades of experience in coaching people though a wide spectrum of chronic and acute pain challenges.

Shinzen leads meditation retreats in the mindfulness tradition throughout North America, and has helped establish several centers and programs.

SOUNDS TRUE was founded in 1985 with a clear vision: to disseminate spiritual wisdom. Located in Boulder, Colorado, Sounds True publishes teaching programs that are designed to educate, uplift, and inspire. With more than 600 titles available, we work with many of the leading spiritual teachers, thinkers, healers, and visionary artists of our time.

For a free catalog, or for more information on audio programs by Shinzen Young, please contact Sounds True via the World Wide Web at www.soundstrue.com, call us toll free at 800-333-9185, or write

The Sounds True Catalog
PO Box 8010
Boulder, CO 80306

CD SESSIONS